The Key to a Flatter Stomach

Boat Pose Workouts for
Defined Abs

Helen Talbott

Disclaimer

The information contained in this book, including text, illustrations, and exercises, is intended for educational and informational purposes only. It is not intended to be a substitute for professional medical advice, diagnosis, or treatment. Always consult with a qualified healthcare professional before starting any new exercise program or making any changes to your diet.

Please be advised:

- Physical Activity Risks: Exercise can inherently carry risks of injury. By participating in the exercises described in this book, you acknowledge and accept these risks. It is strongly recommended that you consult with a healthcare professional before starting any new exercise program, especially if you have any pre-existing medical conditions or injuries.

- Dietary Advice: Any dietary advice offered in this book is for general information only and should not be taken as a substitute for personalized nutritional guidance from a qualified dietitian or other healthcare professional. Your individual needs may vary depending on your health, activity level, and other factors.
- Results Not Guaranteed: The results of the exercise and dietary programs described in this book may vary depending on individual factors and commitment to the program. The author and publisher make no guarantees or warranties regarding the outcomes you may achieve.
- Limitation of Liability: The author and publisher disclaim any liability for any injuries, losses, or damages arising from the use of the information contained in this book. You agree to

assume all risks associated with the use
of this information.

Table of contents

About the author

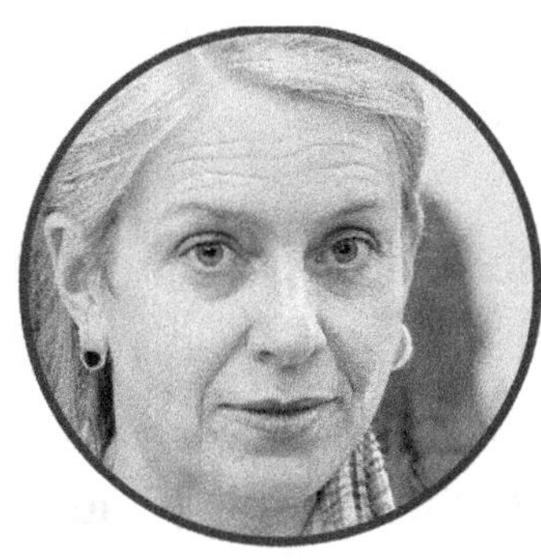

Helen Talbott isn't your average fitness personality. Forget fad diets and grueling cardio sessions. Helen believes in unlocking the power within your own body, using targeted exercises like the boat pose to achieve defined abs and a flatter stomach.

More than just a fitness instructor:

With a background in [sports science, physical therapy, yoga, etc.], Helen's passion goes beyond mere exercise. She understands the intricate relationship between mind, body, and movement. Her approach is holistic, emphasizing the importance of proper form, mindful practice, and self-compassion.

Your journey to sculpted abs starts here:

Helen's book, The Key to a Flatter Stomach: Boat Pose Workouts for Defined Abs, isn't just a collection of exercises. It's a personalized roadmap to success. You'll discover:

- The science behind the boat pose: Why it's the ultimate core-sculpting exercise and how it fits into your overall fitness goals.
- Variations for every level: Whether you're a beginner or a seasoned fitness enthusiast, Helen provides modifications and progressions to keep you challenged and motivated.
- Holistic fitness tips: Learn about nutrition, mindfulness, and self-care practices that contribute to a healthy and sustainable lifestyle.
- Motivational guidance: Helen's warm, encouraging voice will guide you every step of the way, celebrating your victories and supporting you through challenges.

More than just a book, it's a community:

Join Helen's online community where you can connect with other fitness enthusiasts, share your progress, and get personalized support. Ask questions, participate in challenges, and be inspired by others on their journeys to stronger, healthier bodies.

Ready to unlock your core potential?

Dive into Helen's world and discover the transformative power of the boat pose. With her expert guidance and supportive community, you'll achieve a flatter stomach, defined abs, and a newfound confidence in your own body.

Introduction

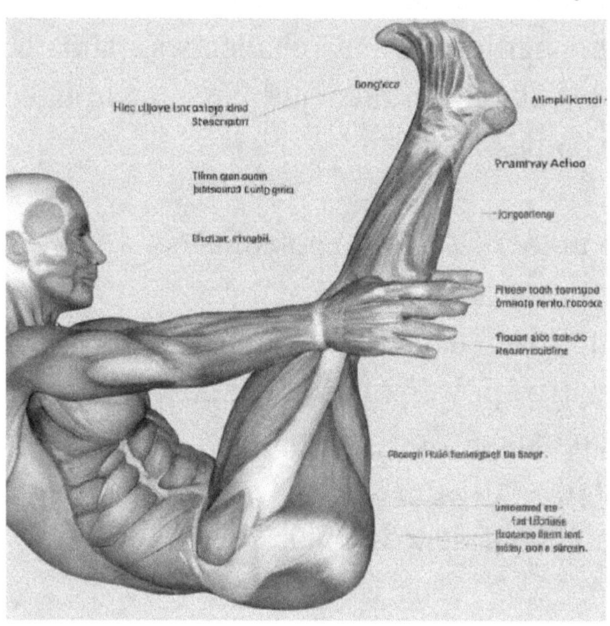

Have you ever gazed longingly at toned abs on magazine covers, dreaming of a flatter stomach and a stronger core? You're not alone! But what if I told you the answer might lie not in endless crunches or grueling fad diets, but in a timeless pose known as Navasana, or the boat pose?

For years, the boat pose has been a secret weapon of yogis and fitness enthusiasts alike. This deceptively simple posture targets and strengthens your core muscles, building a foundation for a flatter stomach, improved posture, and a stronger, more confident you.

But where do you start? Mastering the boat pose and incorporating it into an effective workout routine can be daunting. That's where I come in. As Helen Talbott, a lifelong fitness advocate and your guide on this journey, I'm here to demystify the boat pose and unlock its incredible potential for your core.

In this book, "The Key to a Flatter Stomach: Boat Pose Workouts for Defined Abs," you'll discover:

- The magic of Navasana: Explore the anatomy of the core and how the boat pose specifically targets and

strengthens these muscles, leading to a
flatter stomach and a stronger core.
- Mastering the form: Forget wobbly
  starts and frustrating adjustments. My
  clear instructions and step-by-step
  guides, complete with illustrations, will
  equip you with the perfect boat pose
  technique.
- Tailored workouts: Whether you're a
  beginner just starting out or a seasoned
  exerciser ready for a challenge, I've
  crafted progressive workout programs
  designed to fit your fitness level and
  goals.
- Beyond the boat: Dive deeper into core
  engagement techniques, discover
  variations to keep your workouts
  exciting, and explore lifestyle habits
  that complement your journey.

Forget endless crunches and restrictive diets.
Embrace the power of the boat pose! This

book is your roadmap to a flatter stomach, a stronger core, and a newfound confidence that radiates from the inside out. Are you ready to set sail on your Navasana journey? Join me, and let's unlock your sculpted dreams together!

What is the boat pose and its benefits for a flatter stomach

The boat pose, also known as Navasana, is a yoga posture that engages and strengthens your core muscles, contributing to a flatter stomach in several ways:

Targeting Core Muscles: The boat pose directly targets various core muscles, including the rectus abdominis (six-pack muscles), transverse abdominis (deeper abdominal muscle), and obliques (muscles on the sides of your abdomen). By strengthening these muscles, you create a tighter core, which pulls your stomach in and gives a flatter appearance.

Improved Posture: A strong core improves your overall posture, which can make your stomach appear flatter. Good posture naturally pulls your shoulders back and engages your core, holding your stomach in a more toned position.

Reduced Bloating: Strengthening your core muscles can improve digestion and help reduce bloating, which can contribute to a protruding stomach. The boat pose also massages internal organs, potentially promoting better digestive flow.

Increased Metabolism: Core strength plays a role in your metabolism, and building a stronger core can slightly increase your metabolic rate. This means you burn more calories throughout the day, which can aid in weight management and contribute to a flatter stomach.

Important Note: While the boat pose offers benefits for core strength and potentially a flatter stomach, it's not a magic bullet for weight loss. Achieving a flat stomach requires a combination of healthy eating, regular exercise, and addressing underlying factors like stress and sleep.

Here are some additional benefits of the boat pose:

- Back Strength: The boat pose strengthens your back muscles, which improves posture and prevents back pain.
- Balance and Coordination: This pose challenges your balance and coordination, enhancing overall agility and stability.

- Mood and Energy: Regularly practicing the boat pose can improve mood and energy levels due to increased blood flow and circulation.

Remember, consistency is key. Regular practice of the boat pose, combined with a healthy lifestyle, can contribute to a stronger core, improved posture, and potentially a flatter stomach

Overview of the workout programs and how to use this book.

Get Ready to Unfold Your Core Potential: An Overview of Your Boat Pose Journey

Welcome back to your Navasana adventure! Now that you've delved into the wonders of the boat pose, let's explore the exciting workout programs waiting for you within these pages. Whether you're a complete beginner or a seasoned athlete, there's a path specifically designed to guide you towards your core goals.

The Roadmap to Success:

This book offers three progressive workout programs:

- The 4-Week Beginner Program: This gentle introduction guides you through the fundamentals of the boat pose, building proper form and core engagement alongside beginner-friendly variations.
- The 6-Week Intermediate Program: Once you've mastered the basics, this program elevates your workouts with dynamic variations, longer holds, and additional core exercises to challenge your growing strength.
- The 8-Week Advanced Program: Ready to push your limits? This program unleashes advanced boat pose

variations, dynamic challenges, and longer, more intense workouts to sculpt your core like never before.

Choosing Your Path:

To find your perfect program, consider your current fitness level:

- Beginner: If you're new to exercise or haven't mastered the boat pose, start with the 4-week program.
- Intermediate: Have you been exercising regularly and feel comfortable with basic core exercises? Dive into the 6-week program.
- Advanced: Are you an experienced exerciser seeking a core challenge? The 8-week program is designed for you.

How to Use This Book:

Each program provides:

- Daily workout routines: Detailed instructions, illustrations, and modifications ensure you perform each exercise safely and effectively.
- Progression plans: Gradually increase intensity and duration as you progress through the weeks.
- Tips and troubleshooting: Address common challenges and maximize your results.

Beyond the Workouts:

This book goes beyond just exercises. You'll also discover:

- Nutritional guidelines: Learn how to fuel your body for optimal core development and overall health.
- Lifestyle tips: Explore how sleep, stress management, and hydration impact your core and fitness journey.

Remember: Consistency is key. Commit to regularly practicing your chosen program, listen to your body, and take rest days when needed. Celebrate your progress along the way, and enjoy the empowering journey towards a stronger, flatter stomach and a confident you!

I'm here to guide you every step of the way. Grab your mat, set your intention, and let's unfold your core potential with the power of Navasana!

Chapter 1

Unveiling Your Core's Powerhouse - How the Boat Pose Works Wonders

Welcome to the first chapter of your Navasana exploration! Before we dive into the pose itself, let's embark on a fascinating journey to understand the core we aim to strengthen. Buckle up, as we dissect the anatomy and uncover the magic behind the boat pose's impact on your midsection.

Demystifying the Core:

Forget the six-pack myth! The core is an interconnected network of muscles deeper than just the "abs." It forms a crucial stabilizing and powerhouse around your torso, playing a vital role in:

- Posture: A strong core supports proper alignment, preventing back pain and improving overall well-being.
- Movement: Core muscles facilitate everything from everyday activities like bending to athletic performance.
- Stability: They act as your internal corset, supporting your spine and organs for optimal function.

Key Players in the Core Drama:

Now, let's meet the core muscles that the boat pose specifically targets:

- Rectus abdominis: The infamous "six-pack," responsible for trunk flexion and pulling your navel towards your spine.
- Transverse abdominis: This deeper muscle acts like a corset, drawing your belly in and enhancing stability.

- Obliques: Located on the sides of your abdomen, obliques assist in twisting and bending movements.
- Hip flexors: These muscles connect your pelvis to your legs and are engaged during the boat pose's leg lift.

The Boat Pose - Unleashing Core Strength:

Now, imagine activating all these powerhouse muscles simultaneously! That's exactly what the boat pose does. By lifting your torso and legs off the ground, you:

- Contract your rectus abdominis: Pulling your navel inwards, engaging your "six-pack."
- Activate your transverse abdominis: Like a natural girdle, it draws your belly in and strengthens your core foundation.

- Work your obliques: Maintaining balance engages these muscles as you hold the pose.
- Challenge your hip flexors: Keeping your legs raised keeps these muscles active, contributing to core stability.

Beyond the Abs:

Remember, the boat pose isn't just about aesthetics. It offers a plethora of benefits, including:

- Back strengthening: Improved posture and reduced risk of back pain.
- Improved balance and coordination: Enhanced agility and overall stability.
- Increased metabolism: Potential boost in calorie burning for weight management.
- Enhanced mood and energy: Improved blood flow and circulation can elevate your mood and energy levels.

Ready to Unlock Your Core Potential?

The boat pose awaits, ready to unveil the true power within your core. In the next chapter, we'll delve into mastering the proper form and technique, ensuring you reap the full benefits of this amazing pose. Get ready to take your fitness journey to a whole new level with the magic of Navasana!

Chapter 2

Mastering the Boat Pose Technique - Navigate Your Way to Core Bliss

Welcome back, Navasana adventurer! Now that you understand the core muscle orchestra the boat pose conducts, let's dive into the practicalities of mastering this powerful posture. Remember, proper form is crucial for maximizing results and preventing injury. So, grab your mat, and let's embark on this technique journey together!

Setting the Stage for Success:

Before launching into your first boat pose, ensure a safe and comfortable environment:

- Choose a non-slip yoga mat: This provides stability and prevents slipping.

- Warm up your body: Gentle stretches and light cardio prepare your muscles for the pose.
- Listen to your body: Respect your limitations and modify the pose as needed.

From Land to Boat:

Now, let's break down the boat pose step-by-step:

1. Begin seated: Sit on your mat with knees bent, feet flat on the floor, and spine tall. Engage your core by drawing your belly button towards your spine.
2. Lean back: Gently lean back, balancing on your sitting bones. Engage your core to prevent collapsing onto your back.
3. Lift your legs: Extend both legs straight out in front of you, toes pointed. If this

is challenging, keep your knees slightly
bent initially.

4. Reach forward (optional): Extend your
   arms forward, parallel to the floor,
   fingers reaching towards outstretched
   toes. Keep your back straight and avoid
   hunching.
5. Engage your core: Pull your navel in
   towards your spine, drawing your
   lower ribs down. Imagine zipping up a
   tight corset around your torso.
6. Hold: Maintain the pose for as long as
   you can comfortably, breathing steadily
   and deeply. Aim for 5-10 breaths
   initially, gradually increasing over
   time.
7. Release: Gently lower your legs back
   down to the floor, one at a time. Rest
   for a few breaths before repeating.

Pro Tips for Smooth Sailing:

- Maintain a flat back: Don't hunch your shoulders or round your lower back. Engage your core to keep your spine straight.
- Gaze at your toes: This helps maintain proper neck alignment and prevents straining your gaze.
- Focus on your breath: Breathe deeply and rhythmically throughout the pose to ensure sufficient oxygen flow and maintain focus.
- Modify as needed: If keeping your legs straight is challenging, bend your knees slightly or keep them on the floor with feet hip-width apart.
- Listen to your body: Don't push yourself beyond your limits. If you experience pain, stop the pose and consult a healthcare professional.

Variations to Spice Up Your Practice:

Once you've mastered the basic boat pose, feel free to explore these variations:

- Arm variations: Try raising your arms straight overhead, keeping them alongside your ears.
- Leg variations: Once comfortable, lift one leg at a time while keeping the other extended.
- Hip variations: If balance allows, perform the pose with legs crossed at the ankles.

Embrace the Journey:

Remember, mastering the boat pose takes time and practice. Be patient, celebrate your progress, and enjoy the journey of strengthening your core and sculpting your midsection.

In the next chapter, we'll delve into core engagement principles, helping you

maximize the effectiveness of your boat pose
practice and unlock your full potential!

Are you ready to set sail on your Navasana
adventure? Let's go!

Chapter 3

Avoiding the Rocky Shores - Common Mistakes in the Boat Pose and How to Navigate Them

Welcome back, Navasana voyager! Now that you've mastered the basic form of the boat pose, let's navigate the common pitfalls that can hinder your progress. By understanding and correcting these mistakes, you'll ensure a safe and effective practice, maximizing the benefits of this powerful pose.

Mistake 1: Hunching Your Back

This not only looks incorrect but can also strain your lower back. Remember to keep your spine long and engaged, as if drawing your belly button towards your spine.

Imagine your torso forming a straight line from your shoulders to your hips.

Correction: Engage your core muscles firmly, especially your transverse abdominis. Lift your chest slightly away from your thighs, maintaining a long neck and avoiding straining your chin towards your chest.

Mistake 2: Letting Your Legs Drop

Keeping your legs straight and lifted is crucial for core engagement. Avoid letting them sag towards the floor or wobble excessively.

Correction: Focus on pulling your lower belly in and upwards. Engage your quadriceps and hamstrings to straighten your legs firmly. If this is challenging initially, bend your knees slightly and gradually work towards full extension.

Mistake 3: Forgetting to Breathe

Holding your breath during the pose can deprive your muscles of oxygen, leading to discomfort and reducing your ability to hold the pose for longer.

Correction: Breathe deeply and rhythmically throughout the pose. Inhale as you lean back and exhale as you lower your legs. Focus on expanding your ribcage rather than your shoulders.

Mistake 4: Overlooking Body Alignment

Your body should form a V-shape, with your torso and legs forming two angled lines meeting at your hips. Ensure your shoulders aren't rounded forward or your neck strained.

Correction: Maintain a long neck and gaze softly at your toes or slightly forward. Keep your shoulders relaxed and away from your ears. Engage your core to maintain proper alignment.

Mistake 5: Pushing Beyond Your Limits

Respect your body's limitations. Don't force yourself to stay in the pose longer than comfortable or attempt advanced variations before mastering the basics.

Correction: Listen to your body. If you experience pain, stop the pose and rest. Start with shorter holds and gradually increase duration as your strength improves. Choose beginner-friendly modifications instead of pushing beyond your limits.

Remember: Consistency and proper form are key to safe and effective practice. Celebrate your progress, embrace the journey, and don't be afraid to modify the pose as needed. With dedication and awareness, you'll navigate the boat pose like a seasoned yogi, reaping the

full benefits of this powerful
core-strengthening posture!

In the next chapter, we'll delve into core
engagement principles, further enhancing
your practice and unlocking your full core
potential. Stay tuned!

Chapter 4

Core Engagement Principles for Enhanced Boat Pose Practice

Welcome back, Navasana adventurer! Having conquered the basic form and navigated common pitfalls, we now dive deeper into the heart of the pose: core engagement. By mastering these principles, you'll transform your boat pose from simply holding a position to a powerful core workout, maximizing results and unlocking your full potential.

The Core of the Matter:

Core engagement isn't just about crunching your abs. It's about activating all your core muscles synergistically, creating a stable and

strong foundation for movement. The boat
pose specifically targets these key muscles:

- Rectus abdominis: "Six-pack" for trunk
  flexion and drawing your navel in.

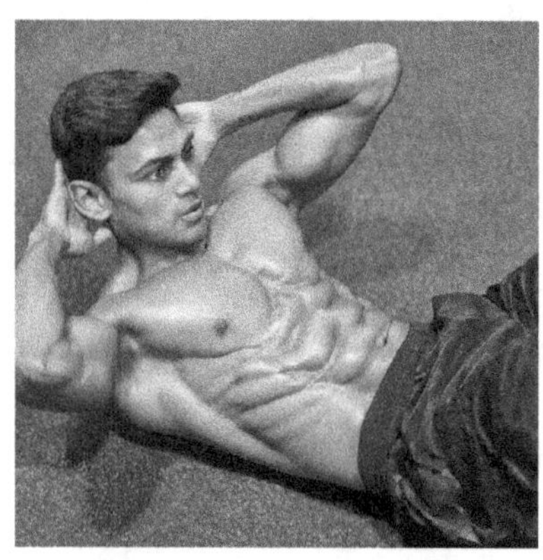

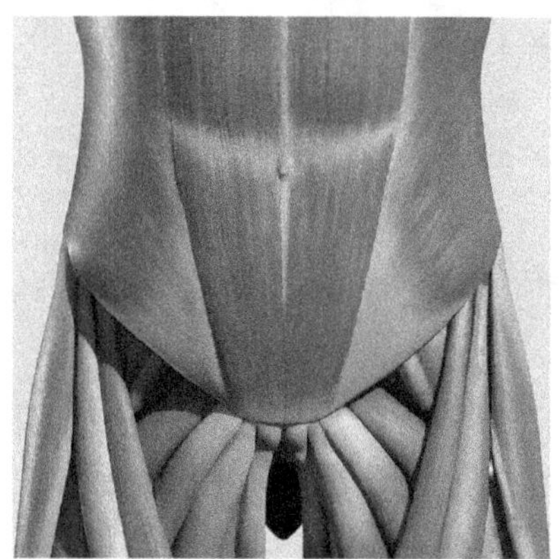

- Transverse abdominis: Deeper muscle like a natural girdle, pulling your belly in and stabilizing your core.
- Obliques: Muscles on your sides for twisting and bending movements.

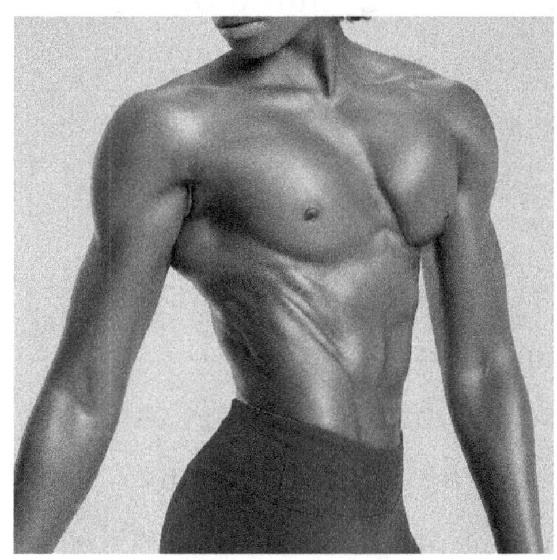

Unlocking the Magic:

Now, let's explore core engagement principles specifically for the boat pose:

1. Breathe Deeply and Actively:

- Don't hold your breath! Inhale deeply
  as you lean back, expanding your
  ribcage.
- Exhale slowly as you lower your legs,
  drawing your belly button inwards.
- Maintain a steady, rhythmic breath
  throughout the pose.

2. Find Your "Draw In":

- Imagine zipping up a tight corset
  around your torso.
- Pull your belly button inwards towards
  your spine, engaging your transverse
  abdominis.
- This deep engagement stabilizes your
  core and protects your lower back.

3. Engage Your Lower Back:

- Don't arch your lower back excessively.

- Instead, imagine tilting your pelvis slightly inwards, tucking your tailbone under.
- This engages your lower core muscles and prevents strain on your back.

4. Activate Your "Inner Thighs":

- Draw your thighs slightly inwards, as if squeezing a ball between them.
- This engages your inner thigh muscles, stabilizing your hips and improving core engagement.

5. Focus on Connection:

- Feel your core muscles working together throughout the pose.
- Imagine your core pulling everything inwards and upwards, creating a strong and stable center.

Beyond the Basics:

Once you've mastered these core engagement
principles, explore advanced techniques:

- Isometric holds: Briefly contract your
  core muscles while holding the pose for
  an extra challenge.
- Pulses: Perform small leg pulses up and
  down while maintaining core
  engagement.
- Dynamic variations: Try lowering and
  lifting one leg at a time or changing
  arm positions.

Remember:

- Consistency is key. Regular practice
  builds core strength and improves your
  boat pose over time.
- Listen to your body. Take breaks and
  choose modifications if needed.
- Enjoy the journey! The boat pose is a
  powerful tool for core strength,
  stability, and even improved mood.

In the next chapter, we'll dive into different workout programs tailored to your fitness level, helping you chart your personal Navasana journey. Get ready to unleash your core potential!

Chapter 5

Boat Pose Workout Programs for Defined Abs

Welcome back, Navasana warrior! Now that you've mastered the art of core engagement, it's time to put your knowledge into action with targeted workout programs designed to sculpt your abs and strengthen your core. Remember, consistency is key, so choose a program that suits your current fitness level and gradually progress as you get stronger.

The Roadmap to Success:

This book offers three progressive workout programs, each designed to guide you on your core-strengthening journey:

- The 4-Week Beginner Program: This gentle introduction focuses on mastering the basic boat pose form with clear instructions, modifications, and progressions.
- The 6-Week Intermediate Program: Once you've established a solid foundation, this program challenges you with dynamic variations, longer holds, and additional core exercises.

The 8-Week Advanced Program: Ready to push your limits? This program incorporates advanced boat pose variations, dynamic challenges, and longer, more intense workouts to truly test your core strength and endurance.

Choosing Your Path:

To find your perfect program, consider your current fitness level:

- Beginner: If you're new to exercise or haven't mastered the boat pose, start with the 4-week program.
- Intermediate: Have you been exercising regularly and feel comfortable with basic core exercises? Dive into the 6-week program.
- Advanced: Are you an experienced exerciser seeking a core challenge? The 8-week program is designed for you.

Remember: Consistency is key. Commit to regularly practicing your chosen program, listen to your body, and take rest days when needed. Celebrate your progress along the way, and enjoy the empowering journey towards a stronger, flatter stomach and a confident you!

General Guidelines:

Before you embark on your workout journey, remember these general tips:

- Warm up: Prepare your body with 5-10 minutes of light cardio and dynamic stretches.
- Cool down: Gently stretch your core and major muscle groups after each workout.
- Listen to your body: Don't push yourself beyond your limits. Take breaks, modify exercises as needed, and stop if you experience pain.
- Focus on form: Proper technique is crucial for maximizing results and preventing injury.
- Breathe deeply: Maintain steady, rhythmic breaths throughout each exercise.
- Hydrate: Drink plenty of water before, during, and after your workouts.

Sample Workout Routines:

Here are sample workout routines from each program to give you a taste of what's to come:

Beginner Program:

- Day 1: 3 sets of 10-second boat pose holds, 3 sets of 15 knee raises, 3 sets of 10 plank variations.
- Day 2: 3 sets of 15-second boat pose holds, 3 sets of 20 bicycle crunches, 3 sets of 12 side plank holds per side.
- Day 3: Rest or active recovery (yoga, walking).

Intermediate Program:

- Day 1: 3 sets of 20-second boat pose holds, 3 sets of 25 mountain climbers, 3 sets of 15 Russian twists per side.
- Day 2: 3 sets of 30-second boat pose holds with leg pulses, 3 sets of 30

flutter kicks, 3 sets of 10 hollow body holds.

- Day 3: 3 sets of 40-second boat pose holds with arm variations, 3 sets of 20 V-ups, 3 sets of 15 side plank hip dips per side.

Advanced Program:

- Day 1: 3 sets of 60-second boat pose holds with variations, 3 sets of 30 hanging leg raises, 3 sets of 20 ab wheel rollouts.
- Day 2: 3 sets of 60-second boat pose holds with single-leg pulses, 3 sets of 30 alternating leg raises, 3 sets of 15 dragon flags.
- Day 3: 3 sets of 60-second boat pose holds with dynamic movements, 3 sets of

Sample Daily Workout Routines for Each Program

Remember: These are just examples, and you can adjust them based on your fitness level and preferences. Always listen to your body and modify exercises as needed.

Warm-up (5-10 minutes):

- Light cardio: Jumping jacks, jogging in place, jumping rope (optional)

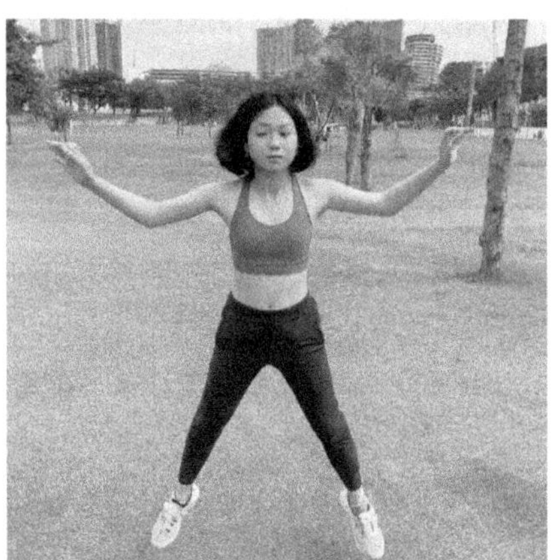

- Dynamic stretches: Arm circles, torso twists, leg swings, lunges with arm raises

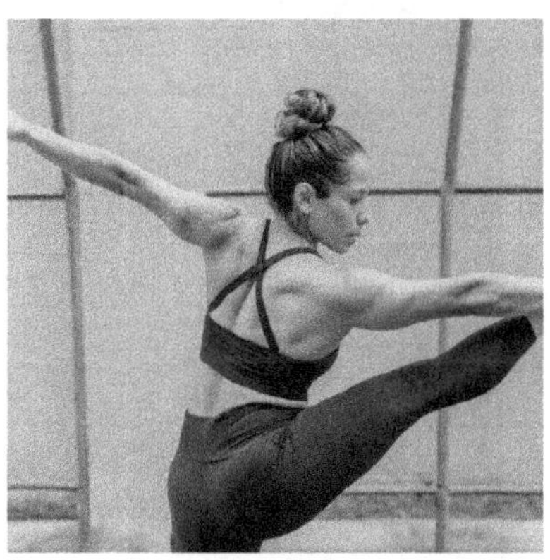

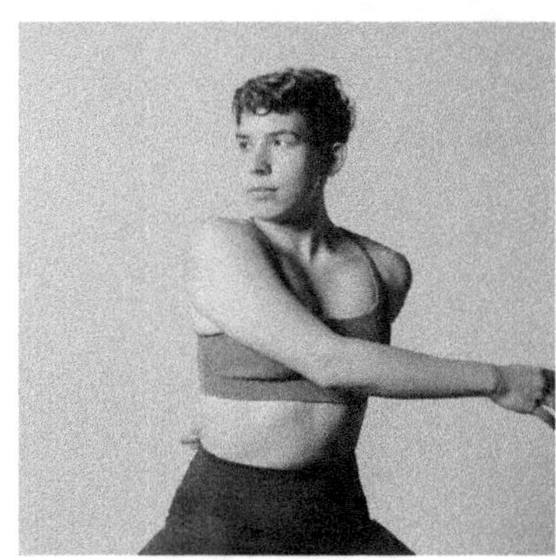

Beginner Program (Day 1):

Focus: Building core strength and proper
boat pose form.

1. Modified Boat Pose (3 sets of 10-15
seconds each):

- Lie on your back with knees bent, feet
  flat on the floor.
- Engage your core and lift your upper
  body and legs off the ground, reaching
  fingertips towards toes.
- Hold for a few seconds, then slowly
  lower back down.
- Modification: Keep knees bent
  throughout if needed.

2. Knee Raises (3 sets of 15-20 repetitions
each):

- Lie on your back with knees bent and
  feet flat on the floor.
- Place your hands behind your head,
  elbows out.

- Engage your core and lift your shoulders and upper back off the ground, bringing your knees towards your chest.
- Lower back down with control.

3. Plank Variations (3 sets of 10-12 repetitions each):

- Start in a high plank position on your hands and forearms, body forming a straight line from head to heels.
- Hold for a few seconds, then try a side plank on each side for a few seconds each.
- Modification: Plank on your knees if needed.

Cool-down (5-10 minutes):

- Gentle stretches: Cat-cow, hamstring stretches, quad stretches, chest openers

Intermediate Program (Day 2):

Focus: Challenging core muscles with dynamic variations and longer holds.

1. Boat Pose with Leg Pulses (3 sets of 30 seconds each):

- Perform the boat pose as described above.
- Once in the hold, pulse one leg up and down for a few seconds, then switch legs.
- Maintain core engagement throughout.

2. Mountain Climbers (3 sets of 25-30 repetitions each):

- Start in a high plank position.
- Bring one knee towards your chest while simultaneously extending the opposite leg back.

- Quickly switch legs, maintaining a fast pace.

3. Russian Twists (3 sets of 15 repetitions per side):

- Sit on the floor with knees bent and feet flat on the ground.
- Lean back slightly, keeping your back straight and core engaged.
- Twist your torso to one side, bringing your hands towards your toes.
- Twist to the other side, keeping your core tight.

Advanced Program (Day 3):

Focus: Pushing limits with advanced variations and intense core strengthening.

1. Boat Pose with Dynamic Movements (3 sets of 60 seconds each):

- Perform the boat pose as described above.
- Try variations like circling your arms overhead, extending one leg at a time, or adding small pulses.
- Maintain core engagement throughout.

2. Hanging Leg Raises (3 sets of 30 repetitions each):

- Hang from a pull-up bar with your palms facing forward.
- Engage your core and lift your straight legs up towards your chest.
- Lower back down with control.
- Modification: Use assisted pull-up bands if needed.

3. Ab Wheel Rollouts (3 sets of 15-20 repetitions each):

- Kneel on a mat with your hands holding an ab wheel in front of you.

- Engage your core and slowly roll the wheel forward, extending your body away from it.
- Roll back towards your knees with control.
- Modification: Start with knees on a higher surface if needed.

Cool-down (5-10 minutes):

- Same as beginner program.

Remember:

- These are just sample routines, and you can modify them to fit your needs.
- Gradually increase the difficulty and duration of your workouts as you get stronger.
- Listen to your body and take rest days when needed.
- Most importantly, enjoy the process and celebrate your progress!

Additional Tips:

- You can find pictures and detailed instructions for each exercise online or in fitness apps.
- Consider investing in a yoga mat and other equipment to enhance your workouts.
- Track your progress in a journal or app to stay motivated.
- Find a workout buddy for added accountability and support.

Chapter 6

Beyond the Exercises - Lifestyle Hacks for a Flatter Stomach and Stronger Core

In your Navasana adventure, remember that achieving a flatter stomach and a stronger core involves more than just exercise. By incorporating healthy lifestyle habits alongside your boat pose workouts, you'll optimize your results and cultivate a holistic approach to well-being.

Nutrition for Core Support:

- Fuel your body: Choose nutrient-rich foods like fruits, vegetables, whole grains, and lean protein to provide your body with the building blocks for strong muscles and optimal health.

- Limit processed foods: Sugary drinks, refined carbohydrates, and unhealthy fats can contribute to inflammation and hinder your progress.
- Mindful eating: Pay attention to hunger cues and avoid overeating. Savor your food and chew thoroughly for better digestion and satiety.
- Hydration is key: Drink plenty of water throughout the day to stay hydrated, aid digestion, and support overall health.

Sleep for Core Recovery:

- Prioritize sleep: Aim for 7-8 hours of quality sleep each night. During sleep, your body repairs and recovers, including your core muscles.
- Create a relaxing bedtime routine: Wind down before bed with calming activities like reading, taking a warm bath, or practicing meditation.

- Optimize your sleep environment:
  Make sure your bedroom is dark, quiet,
  and cool for optimal sleep quality.

Stress Management for a Calmer Core:

- Manage stress: Chronic stress can
  contribute to weight gain and
  negatively impact your core strength.
  Find healthy ways to manage stress,
  such as yoga, meditation, spending
  time in nature, or connecting with
  loved ones.
- Practice mindfulness: Mindfulness
  practices like deep breathing and
  meditation can help you stay present
  and manage stress effectively.
- Identify and address stress triggers:
  Recognizing what triggers your stress
  can help you develop coping
  mechanisms to avoid negative impacts.

Beyond the Body:

- Stay motivated: Surround yourself with supportive people who encourage your fitness journey. Set realistic goals and celebrate your progress along the way.
- Find activities you enjoy: Exercise shouldn't feel like a chore. Explore different activities like dancing, swimming, or hiking to find workouts you enjoy and can stick with.
- Listen to your body: Don't push yourself beyond your limits. Take rest days when needed and respect your body's signals.

Remember, consistency is key. Integrate these lifestyle tips into your routine alongside your dedicated boat pose workouts, and witness the transformative power of a holistic approach to achieving a flatter stomach, a stronger core, and a healthier, happier you!

In the next chapter, we'll wrap up your Navasana journey with a summary, key takeaways, and motivational tips to keep you inspired on your path to core strength and well-being. Stay tuned!

The 4-Week Beginner Program: Your Gateway to a Stronger Core

Welcome to the heart of your beginner journey! This 4-week program gently introduces you to the boat pose and lays the foundation for core strength with clear instructions, modifications, and progressions. Remember, consistency is key, so commit to regular practice and celebrate your progress every step of the way.

Warm-up (5-10 minutes):

- Light cardio: Get your blood pumping with jumping jacks, jogging in place, or jumping rope (optional).
- Dynamic stretches: Prepare your muscles with arm circles, torso twists, leg swings, and lunges with arm raises.

Workout Structure:

This program follows a 3-day per week structure, with each day focusing on different core exercises. Rest or engage in active recovery (walking, yoga) on other days.

Week 1:

Day 1: Core Activation & Boat Pose Introduction

- Plank: Hold a high plank for 30 seconds, then repeat 3 times. Modification: Plank on your knees.
- Bird-Dog: Extend one arm and opposite leg simultaneously, hold for 5 seconds, then switch sides. Repeat 10 times each side.
- Modified Boat Pose: Lie on your back with knees bent, lift upper body and legs slightly off the ground, reaching

fingertips towards toes. Hold for 5
seconds, then lower. Repeat 10 times.

Day 2: Lower Body & Core Integration

- Squats: Perform 15 bodyweight squats,
  focusing on engaging your core.
- Lunges: Do 10 lunges on each leg,
  maintaining good posture and core
  engagement.
- Glute Bridges: Lie on your back with
  knees bent, lift your hips off the
  ground, squeezing your glutes. Hold
  for 5 seconds, then lower. Repeat 15
  times.

Day 3: Rest & Active Recovery

Give your body time to recover with gentle
activities like walking, yoga, or stretching.

Week 2:

Day 1: Progressed Boat Pose & Core
Challenges

- High Plank: Hold a high plank for 45
  seconds, then repeat 3 times.
  Modification: Lower plank on your
  forearms if needed.
- Side Plank: Hold a side plank on each
  side for 30 seconds each. Modification:
  Plank on your knees with your hips
  lifted slightly.
- Boat Pose with Leg Lifts: Perform the
  modified boat pose, then lift one leg at
  a time for 5 seconds each. Repeat 10
  times per leg.

Day 2: Cardio & Core Combo

- Jumping Jacks: Perform 3 sets of 30
  jumping jacks, focusing on core
  engagement with each jump.

- Mountain Climbers: Do 3 sets of 20
  mountain climbers, maintaining a fast
  pace and strong core activation.
- Russian Twists: Sit on the floor with
  knees bent, lean back slightly, and twist
  your torso from side to side, touching
  the ground with your hands. Do 3 sets
  of 15 repetitions per side.

Day 3: Rest & Active Recovery

Enjoy a rest day or incorporate light activities
for recovery.

Weeks 3 & 4:

Gradually increase the duration and intensity
of your exercises while maintaining proper
form. Introduce new variations like boat pose
holds with arm raises or leg pulses. Feel free
to add additional core exercises like crunches
or bicycle kicks to your routines.

Remember:

- Listen to your body and take rest days when needed.
- Modify exercises as needed to ensure proper form and avoid injury.
- Celebrate your progress, no matter how small!

Bonus Tips:

- Track your progress in a journal or app to stay motivated.
- Find a workout buddy for accountability and support.
- Invest in a yoga mat for added comfort and stability.
- Most importantly, have fun and enjoy the process of strengthening your core!

With dedication and consistency, this 4-week program will set you on the path to a stronger core, improved posture, and better overall well-being. Remember, the journey is just as important as the destination, so embrace every step and enjoy the empowering experience of building your core strength!

The 6-Week Intermediate Program

Embark on Your Core Strengthening Adventure

Ready to elevate your core training? The 6-week intermediate program awaits, pushing you beyond the basics and sculpting a stronger, more defined core with dynamic variations, longer holds, and advanced exercises. Remember, consistency and controlled execution are key to unlocking your full potential!

Warm-up (5-10 minutes):

- Light cardio: Get your blood pumping with jumping jacks, jogging in place, or a quick burst of jumping rope (optional).

- Dynamic stretches: Prepare your muscles with arm circles, torso twists, leg swings, and lunges with arm raises.

Workout Structure:

This program follows a 3-day per week structure, targeting different core aspects each day. Rest or engage in active recovery (yoga, swimming) on other days.

Week 1:

Day 1: Core Activation & Dynamic Boat Pose Variations

- Hollow Body Hold: Hold a hollow body position for 30 seconds, focusing on drawing your navel in and engaging your core. Repeat 3 times.
- Side Plank with Hip Dips: Hold a side plank on each side for 30 seconds, with

controlled dips of your hips towards the ground. Repeat 10 times per side.

- Boat Pose with Arm Circles: Perform the boat pose while making small circles with your arms overhead. Hold for 20 seconds, repeat 3 times.

Day 2: Lower Body & Core Integration with Intensity

- Squats with Overhead Press: Perform 12 squats while holding light weights overhead, maintaining core engagement. Repeat 3 sets.
- Jump Squats: Do 3 sets of 15 jump squats, landing softly and engaging your core with each jump.
- Glute Bridges with Single Leg Lifts: Lie on your back, lift your hips, extend one leg straight up, and hold for 5 seconds. Repeat 10 times per leg.

Day 3: Rest & Active Recovery

Listen to your body and allow your muscles to recover with gentle activities.

Week 2:

Day 1: Progressed Boat Pose & Core Challenges

- Anti-Plank: Hold an anti-plank position (face down, forearms on the ground, legs extended back) for 45 seconds, engaging your core. Repeat 3 times.
- Russian Twists with Medicine Ball: Sit with knees bent, lean back slightly, and twist your torso with a medicine ball, touching the ground on each side. Do 3 sets of 15 repetitions per side.
- Boat Pose with Leg Pulses and Arm Raises: Perform the boat pose with alternating leg pulses while raising and lowering your arms. Hold for 30 seconds, repeat 3 times.

Day 2: Cardio & Core Combo with Higher Intensity

- Burpees: Perform 3 sets of 10 burpees, focusing on explosiveness and core engagement throughout the movement.
- Mountain Climbers with Leg Raises: Do 3 sets of 25 mountain climbers, incorporating alternating leg raises for each knee drive.
- Hanging Leg Raises: Hang from a pull-up bar and perform 3 sets of 10 controlled leg raises, keeping your core tight.

Day 3: Rest & Active Recovery

Enjoy a rest day or incorporate light activities like walking or yoga for recovery.

Weeks 3-6:

Gradually increase the duration, intensity, and complexity of your exercises. Introduce advanced variations like boat pose with single-leg holds, plank variations with leg extensions, and dynamic core exercises like ab wheel rollouts. Feel free to add additional exercises that target specific core areas.

Remember:

- Always prioritize proper form over speed or intensity.
- Listen to your body and take rest days when needed.
- Modify exercises as needed to avoid injury.
- Celebrate your progress, no matter how small!

Bonus Tips:

- Track your workouts in a journal or app to monitor progress and stay motivated.

- Find a workout buddy for accountability and support.
- Invest in equipment like weights, a medicine ball, or a pull-up bar to enhance your workouts.
- Most importantly, have fun and enjoy the process of challenging yourself and building a stronger core!

This 6-week intermediate program is your stepping stone to achieving a sculpted core and improved overall fitness. Embrace the journey, stay consistent, and witness the transformative power of dedicated core training!

The 8-Week Advanced Program: Unleash Your Core Potential

Conquer the intermediate level and embark on an advanced 8-week adventure to truly unleash your core potential. This program intensifies the challenge with dynamic variations, longer holds, advanced exercises, and explosive movements, sculpting a defined and powerful core ready for anything. Remember, proper form, controlled execution, and pushing your limits responsibly are key!

Warm-up (5-10 minutes):

- Light cardio: Get your blood pumping with jumping jacks, burpees (optional), or a quick sprint.
- Dynamic stretches: Prepare your muscles with arm circles, torso twists,

leg swings, and lunges with core engagement.

Workout Structure:

This program follows a 3-day per week structure, targeting different core aspects each day. Rest or engage in active recovery (swimming, yoga) on other days.

Week 1:

Day 1: Core Activation & Advanced Boat Pose Variations

- Hollow Body Hold with Leg Raises: Hold a hollow body position for 45 seconds, alternating raising and lowering your legs. Repeat 3 times.
- V-Ups: Lie on your back with legs extended and arms overhead, simultaneously lift your upper body

and legs to form a V-shape. Lower and repeat for 3 sets of 12 repetitions.

- Boat Pose with Windmills: Perform the boat pose while rotating your torso and extending one arm overhead, mimicking a windmill motion. Hold for 15 seconds per side, repeat 3 times.

Day 2: Lower Body & Core Integration with Explosive Power

- Pistol Squats: Perform 3 sets of 10 pistol squats on each leg, focusing on core engagement and balance.
- Box Jumps: Do 3 sets of 8 box jumps (height adjusted to your level), landing softly and engaging your core.
- Glute Bridges with Single Leg Hip Thrusts: Lie on your back, lift your hips, extend one leg straight up, and thrust your hips forward. Repeat 12 times per leg.

Day 3: Rest & Active Recovery

Allow your muscles to recover and refuel for the next challenge.

Week 2:

Day 1: Progressed Boat Pose & Core Challenges with Intensity

- Dragon Flag: Lie on a bench with your back supported and legs extended, lower your body towards the ground while maintaining a straight line and engaging your core. Hold for 5 seconds, repeat 3 times.
- Ab Wheel Rollouts with Leg Extensions: Perform ab wheel rollouts while extending one leg straight out in front of you. Roll out and in for 3 sets of 8 repetitions per leg.
- Boat Pose with Leg Circles: While in the boat pose, make small circles with

one leg extended, then switch. Hold for 30 seconds per side, repeat 3 times.

Day 2: Cardio & Core Combo with Advanced Movements

- Box Jumps with Tuck Jumps: Perform 3 sets of 10 box jumps, adding a tuck jump at the top for explosive core engagement.
- Mountain Climbers with Scissor Kicks: Do 3 sets of 20 mountain climbers, alternating with scissor kicks during each knee drive.
- Hanging Leg Raises with Knee Raises: Hang from a pull-up bar, perform 3 sets of 8 controlled leg raises, followed by 3 sets of 12 knee raises, focusing on core activation throughout.

Day 3: Rest & Active Recovery

Enjoy a rest day or incorporate light activities like walking or yoga for recovery.

Weeks 3-8:

Gradually increase the duration, intensity, and complexity of your exercises. Introduce advanced variations like single-leg boat pose holds with dynamic movements, plank variations with core twists, and advanced core exercises like L-sit holds. Feel free to add challenging exercises that target specific core areas.

Remember:

- Always prioritize proper form over speed or intensity.
- Listen to your body and take rest days when needed.
- Modify exercises as needed to avoid injury.

- Celebrate your progress, no matter how small!

Bonus Tips:

- Track your workouts in a journal or app to monitor progress and stay motivated.
- Find a workout buddy for accountability and support.
- Invest in equipment like weights, a medicine ball, a pull-up bar, and ab wheel to enhance your workouts.
- Most importantly, have fun and challenge yourself while pushing your limits responsibly!

Remember, this 8-week program is a demanding journey, but with dedication and the right approach, you'll sculpt a powerful core and elevate your overall fitness to new heights. Embrace the challenge, stay consistent, and enjoy the ride!

Chapter 7

The Importance of Diet for Core Definition

Building a strong, defined core goes beyond crunches and boat poses. While exercise plays a crucial role, achieving a flatter stomach and visible abs also requires fueling your body with the right nutrients. In this chapter, we'll explore the dietary cornerstones for core definition, helping you make informed choices that complement your workout efforts.

The Power of Food:

Think of your diet as the foundation for your core strength and definition. Just like building a house, you need sturdy materials to create a solid structure. The right foods provide the essential building blocks (protein), energy sources (healthy fats and complex carbohydrates), and recovery tools (vitamins and minerals) your core needs to thrive.

Key Dietary Principles:

- Prioritize Protein: Protein is the cornerstone of muscle building and repair. Aim for 0.8-1 gram of protein per pound of body weight daily. Choose lean protein sources like chicken, fish, beans, lentils, tofu, and low-fat dairy.
- Embrace Healthy Fats: Don't fear fats! Healthy fats like avocados, nuts, seeds, and olive oil aid in nutrient absorption, support cell function, and keep you feeling satiated.
- Choose Complex Carbs: Ditch refined carbohydrates like white bread and pastries. Instead, opt for complex carbs like whole grains, fruits, and

vegetables. They provide sustained energy and fiber, aiding digestion and preventing blood sugar spikes.

- Limit Processed Foods: Processed foods are often packed with unhealthy fats, added sugars, and sodium, hindering your progress. Opt for whole, unprocessed foods whenever possible.
- Stay Hydrated: Water is essential for overall health and core function. Aim for 8 glasses of water daily to flush toxins, aid digestion, and support muscle recovery.

Beyond the Basics:

Remember, these are general guidelines. Tailoring your diet to your individual needs and preferences is crucial. Consider consulting a registered dietitian for personalized advice. Additionally, explore these tips for maximizing your dietary impact:

- Mindful Eating: Pay attention to hunger and fullness cues. Savor your food and avoid mindless snacking.
- Portion Control: Use smaller plates, measure your food, and avoid overeating, even healthy options.
- Meal Planning and Prepping: Planning your meals and prepping healthy snacks can help you stay on track and avoid unhealthy temptations.
- Read Food Labels: Be mindful of hidden sugars and unhealthy fats by checking food labels diligently.

Remember:

Achieving core definition is a journey, not a destination. A balanced diet combined with consistent exercise is the key to success. Embrace healthy eating habits, enjoy nutritious foods, and witness the transformative power of nourishing your body from within!

Next Steps:

In the next chapter, we'll explore additional lifestyle habits that complement your diet and exercise efforts, further optimizing your journey towards a stronger, more defined core.

**Nutritional Guidelines for Fat Loss and
Muscle Building**
Striking the Balance

Achieving both fat loss and muscle building
simultaneously requires a strategic approach
to your diet. It's not just about eating less; it's
about fueling your body with the right
nutrients to optimize both processes. Here are
some key guidelines to remember:

Calories:

- Calorie Deficit for Fat Loss: To lose
  fat, you need to create a calorie deficit,
  meaning you burn more calories than
  you consume. Aim for a moderate
  deficit of 300-500 calories per day to
  avoid losing muscle mass.
- Slight Surplus for Muscle Gain: For
  muscle building, a small calorie surplus
  of 200-300 calories per day is

recommended to provide enough
energy for muscle growth and repair.

Macronutrients:

- Protein: This is the building block of
  muscle! Aim for 0.8-1 gram of protein
  per pound of bodyweight daily. Good
  sources include lean meats, fish, eggs,
  dairy, legumes, and tofu.
- Carbohydrates: These provide energy
  for your workouts and daily activities.
  Choose complex carbs like whole
  grains, fruits, and vegetables, which
  offer fiber and sustained energy. Limit
  refined carbs like white bread and
  sugary drinks.
- Healthy Fats: Don't shy away from
  healthy fats like avocados, nuts, seeds,
  and olive oil. They aid in nutrient
  absorption, hormone production, and
  satiety.

Other Important Nutrients:

- Fiber: Include plenty of fiber-rich foods like fruits, vegetables, and whole grains to aid digestion, keep you feeling full, and manage blood sugar levels.
- Micronutrients: Ensure you're getting enough vitamins and minerals through a balanced diet or consider a multivitamin to support overall health and muscle function.

Additional Tips:

- Spread your protein intake throughout the day: Aim for 20-30 grams of protein at each meal and snack.
- Plan and prepare your meals: This helps you make healthy choices and avoid unhealthy temptations.
- Stay hydrated: Water is essential for all bodily functions, including muscle recovery and nutrient absorption.

- Listen to your body: Pay attention to hunger and fullness cues, and don't restrict yourself unnecessarily.
- Seek professional guidance: Consider consulting a registered dietitian for personalized advice tailored to your specific goals and needs.

Remember, consistency is key. Sticking to these guidelines and making healthy choices most of the time will yield better results than restrictive diets or quick fixes.

Important Note:

While these guidelines provide a starting point, it's crucial to remember that individual needs vary based on factors like age, activity level, and metabolism. Consulting a healthcare professional or registered dietitian is always recommended for personalized advice and to ensure your approach aligns with your health and fitness goals.

Sample Meal Plans and Healthy Recipes for Fat Loss and Muscle Building

Here are two sample meal plans and some healthy recipes to get you started on your journey towards fat loss and muscle building. Remember, these are just examples, and you may need to adjust them based on your individual needs and preferences.

Sample Meal Plan 1 (For Muscle Building):

Breakfast:

- Scrambled eggs with spinach and whole-wheat toast: Eggs are a great source of protein, while spinach provides vitamins and minerals. Whole-wheat toast offers complex carbohydrates for sustained energy.
- Fruit smoothie with protein powder: This provides protein, vitamins, and

minerals, and helps you feel full until lunchtime.

Lunch:

- Grilled chicken breast with brown rice and roasted vegetables: This is a classic muscle-building meal with lean protein, complex carbohydrates, and healthy fats.
- Side salad with vinaigrette dressing: Add some extra fiber and vitamins to your lunch.

Dinner:

- Salmon with quinoa and steamed broccoli: Salmon is rich in omega-3 fatty acids, which are beneficial for overall health and muscle function. Quinoa is a complete protein source, and broccoli provides vitamins and fiber.

Snacks:

- Greek yogurt with fruit and nuts
- Cottage cheese with vegetables
- Hard-boiled eggs
- Trail mix with nuts and seeds

Sample Meal Plan 2 (For Fat Loss):

Breakfast:

- Oats with berries and chia seeds: This is a fiber-rich breakfast that will keep you feeling full until lunchtime. Berries add antioxidants, and chia seeds provide healthy fats and omega-3s.
- Green tea: This helps boost metabolism and aids in digestion.

Lunch:

- Tuna salad sandwich on whole-wheat bread with lettuce and tomato: Tuna is

a lean protein source, and whole-wheat
bread provides complex carbohydrates.
Lettuce and tomato add vitamins and
fiber.

- Vegetable soup: This is a low-calorie
and filling option.

Dinner:

- Lentil soup with whole-wheat bread:
Lentils are a plant-based protein source
rich in fiber. Whole-wheat bread adds
complex carbohydrates.
- Side salad with vinaigrette dressing:
Add some extra fiber and vitamins to
your dinner.

Snacks:

- Apple slices with almond butter
- Carrot sticks with hummus
- Edamame
- Air-popped popcorn

Healthy Recipes:

Here are some quick and easy recipes to try:

- Scrambled Eggs with Spinach and Whole-Wheat Toast: Whisk 2 eggs with a splash of milk and salt and pepper. Sauté spinach in a pan with olive oil. Add the eggs and scramble until cooked through. Serve on whole-wheat toast.
- Grilled Chicken Breast with Brown Rice and Roasted Vegetables: Preheat oven to 400°F. Season chicken breast with salt, pepper, and your favorite spices. Roast for 20-25 minutes, or until cooked through. Cook brown rice according to package instructions. Roast your favorite vegetables (e.g., broccoli, carrots, asparagus) with olive oil, salt, and pepper for 20-25 minutes, or until tender-crisp.

- Salmon with Quinoa and Steamed Broccoli: Preheat oven to 400°F. Season salmon with salt, pepper, and your favorite spices. Roast for 15-20 minutes, or until cooked through. Cook quinoa according to package instructions. Steam broccoli until tender-crisp.
- Oats with Berries and Chia Seeds: Cook oats according to package instructions. Top with berries, chia seeds, and a drizzle of honey or maple syrup (optional).
- Tuna Salad Sandwich on Whole-Wheat Bread with Lettuce and Tomato: Mix canned tuna with mayonnaise, diced celery, onion, and your favorite seasonings. Spread on whole-wheat bread and top with lettuce and tomato.
- Lentil Soup with Whole-Wheat Bread: Sauté onion, garlic, and carrots in a pot with olive oil. Add lentils, vegetable

broth, and your favorite spices. Bring
to a boil, then reduce heat and simmer
for 30 minutes, or until lentils are
tender. Serve with whole-wheat bread.

Remember, these are just a few examples,
and there are endless possibilities for healthy
and delicious meals. Explore different
recipes, ingredients, and cooking methods to
find what you enjoy and fits your needs.
Most importantly, have fun and enjoy the
process!

Chapter 8

Lifestyle Habits for a Flatter Stomach - Beyond Diet and Exercise

In your core-strengthening journey, remember that achieving a flatter stomach and a healthier you goes beyond just diet and exercise. By incorporating healthy lifestyle habits alongside your boat pose workouts and nutritious meals, you'll cultivate a holistic approach to well-being and optimize your results.

Sleep for Core Recovery and Stress Management:

- Prioritize quality sleep: Aim for 7-8 hours of uninterrupted sleep each night. During sleep, your body repairs and recovers, including your core muscles.

- Create a relaxing bedtime routine:
  Wind down before bed with calming
  activities like reading, taking a warm
  bath, or practicing meditation.
- Optimize your sleep environment:
  Ensure your bedroom is dark, quiet,
  and cool for optimal sleep quality.
- Manage stress: Chronic stress can
  contribute to weight gain and hinder
  your progress. Find healthy ways to
  manage stress, such as yoga, spending
  time in nature, or connecting with
  loved ones.

Hydration for Optimal Function:

- Drink plenty of water: Aim for 8
  glasses of water throughout the day to
  stay hydrated, aid digestion, and
  support overall health.
- Limit sugary drinks: Avoid sugary
  beverages like soda, juice, and sports

drinks, which can contribute to weight gain and bloating.

- Choose herbal teas and infused water: Opt for unsweetened herbal teas or water infused with fruits, vegetables, or herbs for added flavor and potential health benefits.

Mindful Eating Habits:

- Practice mindful eating: Pay attention to hunger and fullness cues. Avoid distractions while eating and savor your food thoroughly.
- Don't skip meals: Skipping meals can lead to overeating later. Aim for regular meals and healthy snacks throughout the day to keep your metabolism stable.
- Portion control: Use smaller plates, measure your food, and avoid mindlessly snacking.

Movement Beyond the Gym:

- Stay active throughout the day: Take the stairs instead of the elevator, park farther away, and incorporate short walks or stretches throughout your day.
- Find activities you enjoy: Explore different physical activities like dancing, swimming, hiking, or biking to find workouts you look forward to and can stick with.
- Engage in stress-relieving activities: Exercise releases endorphins, which have mood-boosting and stress-reducing effects. Choose activities you find enjoyable and relaxing.

Additional Tips:

- Limit processed foods: Processed foods are often high in unhealthy fats, added sugars, and sodium, which can contribute to bloating and hinder your progress.

- Manage portion sizes: Be mindful of portion sizes, even for healthy foods. Overeating, regardless of the food choices, can hinder your goals.
- Track your progress: Keeping a journal or using an app to track your progress can help you stay motivated and celebrate your achievements.
- Seek support: Surround yourself with supportive people who encourage your healthy lifestyle choices. Consider joining a fitness group or working with a registered dietitian or personal trainer.

Remember, consistency is key! By incorporating these lifestyle habits into your routine alongside your dedicated exercise and mindful eating, you'll create a sustainable approach to achieving a flatter stomach, a stronger core, and a healthier, happier you!

This concludes your comprehensive guide to achieving a flatter stomach and building a stronger core. Remember, the journey is just as important as the destination, so embrace each step, celebrate your progress, and enjoy the empowering experience of transforming your core and overall well-being!

**The Impact of Sleep, Stress, and
Hydration on Core Definition: Unveiling
the Hidden Players**

While exercise and diet are crucial for core
definition, often overlooked factors like
sleep, stress, and hydration play equally
important roles. Let's delve into their
individual and combined impact:

Sleep:

- Muscle Repair and Recovery: During
  sleep, your body releases growth
  hormone, essential for muscle repair
  and growth. Inadequate sleep hinders
  this process, impacting core definition
  progress.
- Reduced Cortisol Levels: Cortisol, the
  stress hormone, can lead to muscle
  breakdown and fat storage, especially
  around the abdomen. Quality sleep

helps regulate cortisol levels, promoting a leaner core.

- Improved Performance: Sleep deprivation affects energy levels, focus, and coordination, hindering workout performance and impacting core engagement during exercises.

Stress:

- Elevated Cortisol Levels: As mentioned earlier, chronic stress elevates cortisol, leading to muscle breakdown and fat storage around the midsection.
- Increased Cravings: Stress triggers the release of hormones that can increase cravings for sugary and unhealthy foods, hindering your dietary efforts for core definition.
- Disrupted Sleep: Stress can make it difficult to fall asleep and stay asleep, creating a vicious cycle that further

compounds the negative effects on core definition.

Hydration:

- Muscle Function: Dehydration reduces muscle performance and endurance, impacting the effectiveness of your core workouts.
- Digestive Health: Proper hydration promotes efficient digestion, preventing bloating and constipation that can contribute to a less defined core appearance.
- Nutrient Absorption: Water is essential for transporting nutrients to your muscles, including those in your core, optimizing their growth and function.

The Synergistic Effect:

These factors don't operate in isolation. They have a synergistic effect, meaning addressing one can positively impact the others. For example, good sleep helps manage stress, which in turn improves sleep quality and reduces cortisol levels, ultimately aiding core definition.

Optimizing Your Strategy:

- Prioritize quality sleep: Aim for 7-8 hours of uninterrupted sleep each night.
- Develop stress management techniques: Practice yoga, meditation, or deep breathing exercises to manage stress and its negative effects.
- Stay hydrated: Drink plenty of water throughout the day, aiming for 8-10 glasses, and adjust based on your activity level and climate.
- Maintain a balanced diet: Nourish your body with nutrient-rich foods while remaining mindful of portion sizes.
- Engage in regular exercise: Consistent core-focused workouts combined with

cardio strengthen your core muscles
and promote overall fitness.

Remember, achieving core definition is a
journey, not a destination. By addressing
these lifestyle factors alongside your exercise
and diet routine, you create a holistic
approach that optimizes your results and
unlocks the full potential of your
core-strengthening efforts. So, sleep well,
manage stress, stay hydrated, and witness the
transformative power of a well-rounded
approach!

Conclusion

As you turn the final page, remember that this journey wasn't just about achieving a flatter stomach or defined abs. It was about embarking on a path of self-discovery, cultivating strength, and empowering yourself to live a healthier, more confident life.

The boat pose wasn't just an exercise; it was a metaphor for navigating life's challenges with balance and resilience. Through each hold, you built not just core muscle, but also the mental fortitude to overcome obstacles and achieve your goals.

By prioritizing sleep, managing stress, staying hydrated, and making mindful choices, you transcended the physical and embraced a holistic approach to well-being. This newfound awareness will serve you far beyond the realm of fitness, impacting your

energy levels, mood, and overall outlook on
life.

Remember, the journey continues. Keep
exploring, keep challenging yourself, and
most importantly, keep believing in your
ability to achieve anything you set your mind
to.

Here are some concluding thoughts to inspire
you:

- Celebrate your journey: Acknowledge
  the progress you've made, both big and
  small. Be proud of yourself for taking
  this transformative step towards a
  healthier you.
- Embrace the power of community:
  Surround yourself with supportive
  people who share your passion for
  wellness and encourage your continued
  growth.

- Explore new horizons: Don't be afraid to step outside your comfort zone and try new fitness activities, healthy recipes, or personal development practices.
- Make sustainable choices: Remember, true transformation is about long-term habits, not quick fixes. Focus on building healthy routines you can enjoy and maintain for life.
- Never stop learning: The world of health and fitness is constantly evolving. Embrace the opportunity to learn new things, stay curious, and continue to refine your approach.

May your core, both physical and mental, remain strong and empowered as you navigate the exciting journey ahead. Thank you for taking this adventure with me, and remember, the key to a flatter stomach truly lies within the power of your own determination and a holistic approach to well-being.

Boat Pose Workout Log

Columns:

- Date: The date you performed the workout.
- Duration (Seconds): The total time you held the boat pose in seconds. Aim to increase this duration gradually over time.
- Hold Quality: Rate your ability to hold the pose with proper alignment and engagement. "Excellent" means you held the pose with perfect form, while "Needs Work" indicates room for improvement.
- Modifications Used: Indicate whether you used any modifications to make the pose easier, such as using blocks or holding onto a wall.
- Additional Notes: Use this space to record any relevant observations, such as challenges you faced, areas of improvement, or how you felt after the workout.

Tips:

- You can create additional columns to track specific aspects of your boat pose, such as core engagement, leg alignment, or arm position.
- Use different colors or symbols to highlight areas of progress or setbacks.
- Set realistic goals and track your progress over time to stay motivated.

Request for a review

Attention Fitness Bloggers and Reviewers! Unleash the Power of the Boat Pose for a Flatter Stomach

Are you looking for a unique and effective approach to getting defined abs and a flatter stomach? My book, The Key to a Flatter Stomach: Boat Pose Workouts for Defined Abs, offers a revolutionary approach using the often-overlooked but incredibly powerful boat pose.

Why your audience will love this book:

- Science-backed approach: Discover the how and why behind the boat pose's effectiveness, with research-based explanations for its core-sculpting magic.
- No fad diets or grueling cardio: This book focuses on targeted exercises and mindful movement, promoting a sustainable and enjoyable fitness journey.
- Suitable for all levels: Modifications and progressions cater to beginners and seasoned fitness enthusiasts alike, ensuring everyone can achieve results.

- Holistic approach: Goes beyond physical exercise, offering guidance on nutrition, mindfulness, and self-care for a well-rounded approach to health and wellness.
- Motivational and supportive: My encouraging voice guides readers through challenges and celebrates their victories, fostering a positive and sustainable fitness journey.

I'm seeking reviewers who:

- Are passionate about fitness and health.
- Appreciate unique and effective exercise approaches.
- Connect with and resonate with my holistic and encouraging style.
- Have an audience interested in achieving defined abs and a flatter stomach.

What I offer reviewers:

- A complimentary copy of the book in your preferred format (ebook, paperback)
- The chance to make a positive impact on your readers' health and fitness journeys.

I look forward to partnering with you to help unleash
the power of the boat pose for a healthier and
happier audience!

Sincerely,

Helen Talbott